I0119083

GUIDE TEN:
SCALP HEALTH STARTS HERE

From Root to Tip: A Growing Hands Guide for Natural Hair

BY CONSTANCE HUNTER

COPYRIGHT © 2025 BY CONSTANCE HUNTER ALL RIGHTS RESERVED.

No part of this book may be reproduced, distributed, or transmitted in any form or by any means—including photocopying, recording, or other electronic or mechanical methods—without prior written permission from the publisher, except in the case of brief quotations used in critical reviews or other noncommercial purposes permitted by copyright law.

For permissions, inquiries, or additional resources, please contact:

Pre'Vail Natural Hair Salon

www.prevailyournatural.com | prevailyournatural@gmail.com

This book is intended for informational and educational purposes only and should serve as a general guide to understanding and improving natural hair health. While the methods and recommendations provided are based on expertise in natural hair care and trichology, they are not intended to replace professional medical or dermatological advice.

If you are experiencing severe scalp conditions, excessive hair loss, or other persistent issues, it is strongly recommended that you consult a licensed dermatologist or a professional cosmetologist specializing in scalp and hair health. A trained professional can assess underlying causes and provide personalized treatment plans tailored to your specific needs.

By using the information in this book, the reader acknowledges that the author and publisher are not responsible for individual outcomes. Readers should exercise their own discretion when applying the suggested practices.

First Edition: 2025

ISBN:

Paperback: 978-1-968134-00-6

Ebook: 978-1-968134-19-8

Printed in USA

ABOUT THE AUTHOR

As a certified trichologist and natural hair care educator, I specialize in helping individuals discover what's truly possible for their hair—especially when they've been told otherwise.

My passion lies in witnessing transformation—that moment when someone realizes their hair can be healthy, strong, and free. With a deep understanding of the science behind hair and scalp health, I strive to provide clarity, comfort, and actionable solutions. My training equips me to assess and guide care for a wide range of concerns, from common challenges like dandruff and dryness to complex conditions such as alopecia areata, scalp psoriasis, and CCCA.

But my work goes beyond diagnosis or technique. I believe in education, empowerment, and helping clients build routines that nourish their crown from root to tip. This includes learning to read labels, choosing products with purpose, avoiding harmful styling practices, and embracing care that fits their lifestyle and values.

While I offer expert insight from the field of trichology, I'm not a medical doctor. Hair and scalp symptoms can sometimes signal deeper health issues. That's why I encourage a holistic approach—and, when necessary, consulting licensed healthcare professionals for comprehensive support.

In this series, you'll find guidance rooted in science, experience, and care. My hope is that it not only helps you understand your hair better but also love it more, trust it more, and grow with it in ways you never thought possible.

Your hair is not the problem—you just needed the right guide.

DEDICATION

For the one who hides her scalp and suffers in silence.
There's nothing shameful here—only healing, waiting to
begin.

OVERVIEW

A thriving crown starts at the roots. *Scalp Health Starts Here* is your guide to healing and protecting the foundation of your hair: your scalp. Whether you're dealing with flaking, inflammation, hair thinning, or simply want to maintain a healthy environment for growth, this guide offers real answers and long-term relief.

True hair care doesn't start with your strands—it starts beneath them.

SERIES INTRODUCTION

Welcome to *From Root to Tip: A Growing Hands Guide for Natural Hair*

This series was created with one goal in mind: to give you what's been missing—not just products, not just trends, but truth, support, and real guidance for real people who are ready to finally understand and care for their natural hair from the inside out.

For years, we've been taught to manage, fix, or fight our hair. But here, we're doing something different. We're returning to care—not control. To confidence. To consistency. To choice.

Each guide in this series is built as a step in your journey. They can be read in order or on their own, depending on where you are in your process. Whether you're just starting out, rebuilding your relationship with your hair, or deepening your understanding, this space is for you.

I've written these guides from my hands—growing hands that have touched, healed, protected, and restored countless crowns. Now, I offer that care to you.

This isn't just about hair. It's about healing. It's about reclaiming your rhythm, your confidence, and your beauty—from root to tip.

Let's begin.

WHAT YOU WILL LEARN

- How to recognize the symptoms of common scalp conditions

- Causes and triggers of hair loss, inflammation, and sensitivity

- Steps to support regrowth and reduce long-term damage

- When to seek help from dermatologists and trichologists

- How to create a scalp care routine that fits your lifestyle

- Natural and holistic care options: massage, oils, nutrition, and more

WHAT YOU'LL WALK AWAY WITH

- A clearer understanding of your scalp's needs and health

- Practical, gentle methods for soothing and restoring balance

- Confidence in how and when to seek professional support

- A renewed mindset: your healing is possible—and you're not alone

TABLE OF CONTENTS

INTRODUCTION

If your scalp could talk, what would it say? Too often, we focus on length while ignoring the root of the issue. *Scalp Health Starts Here* brings attention back to the place where growth truly begins. You'll learn how to recognize early signs of imbalance, understand common conditions like CCCA, traction alopecia, dermatitis, and psoriasis, and take action with both home care and professional support.

This is the guide for those who need clarity, comfort, and a plan to restore what's been lost—physically and emotionally.

UNDERSTANDING AND ADDRESSING AFRICAN AMERICAN HAIR AND SCALP HEALTH

Introduction

African American hair is characterized by its unique curl patterns, structural differences, and increased fragility compared to other hair types. These attributes require specialized care and understanding to maintain both hair and scalp health. This module explores common issues, underlying causes, diagnostic methods, and effective solutions tailored to African American hair. By addressing cultural practices and scientific insights, we aim to provide a comprehensive guide for individuals seeking to improve hair and scalp health.

Common Hair and Scalp Issues

Central Centrifugal Cicatricial Alopecia (CCCA) is a type of scarring alopecia that primarily affects African American women. This progressive condition begins with hair loss at the crown of the scalp and gradually spreads outward. If left untreated, CCCA can lead to permanent hair follicle destruction due to scarring. Understanding its causes, recognizing symptoms early, and seeking timely treatment are crucial for effective management.

Causes of CCCA

Although the exact cause of CCCA remains unclear, research indicates that multiple factors contribute to its development:

1. Chemical Damage

Frequent use of chemical relaxers, harsh dyes, and straighteners can weaken the hair shaft and scalp, leading to inflammation of the hair follicles. Over time, this inflammation may cause scarring and permanent hair loss.

2. Heat & Mechanical Trauma

- Regular use of flat irons, curling irons, and blow dryers at high temperatures can damage the hair cuticle and scalp.
- Tight hairstyles (e.g., braiding, weaving, cornrows, ponytails) place excessive tension on the follicles, leading to stress and inflammation.

3. Genetic Factors

Studies suggest a hereditary component to CCCA, meaning individuals with a family history of the condition may be more susceptible.

4. Autoimmune & Inflammatory Response

CCCA has been linked to perifollicular inflammation and fibrosis, where the immune system mistakenly attacks hair follicles, resulting in scarring.

5. Nutritional Deficiencies

Deficiencies in essential nutrients, such as iron, vitamin D, and fatty acids, have been associated with an increased risk of hair loss and scalp inflammation.

Symptoms of CCCA

The symptoms of CCCA progress gradually, making early detection crucial.

Early Signs

- **Itching & Burning Sensation** – Tingling or warmth, especially at the crown.
- **Scalp Tenderness & Pain** – Discomfort when touching or styling the hair.

- **Redness & Inflammation** – Signs of active follicular damage.

Progressive Symptoms

- **Hair Thinning at the Crown** – Gradual loss that spreads outward.
- **Perifollicular Scaling & Pustules** – Small bumps or white scaling around hair follicles.
- **Scarring & Shiny Bald Patches** – As follicles are replaced with scar tissue, leading to irreversible baldness.

Solutions & Treatment Options

Managing CCCA requires early intervention and a multifaceted approach, including lifestyle changes, medical treatments, and scalp care.

1. **Early Intervention**

- **Avoid Chemical Relaxers & Heat Tools** – These can worsen inflammation and follicular damage.
- **Choose Low-Manipulation Hairstyles** – Loose twists and protective styles with minimal tension help reduce stress on hair follicles.
- **Use Gentle Shampoos** – Opt for sulfate-free cleansers to protect the scalp's natural moisture barrier.

2. **Medical Treatments**

- **Topical & Injectable Corticosteroids** – Help reduce inflammation and slow scarring.
- **Topical Minoxidil (Rogaine 5%)** – Encourages hair regrowth in areas where follicles are still active.
- **Antibiotics (e.g., Doxycycline, Clindamycin)** – Used to control follicular inflammation.

- **Hydroxychloroquine** – Sometimes prescribed for autoimmune-related scalp conditions.
- **Platelet-Rich Plasma (PRP) Therapy** – Uses growth factors from the patient's blood to stimulate hair follicle regeneration.

3. **Nutritional Support**

- **Iron & Vitamin D Supplements** – Essential for hair growth and follicular health.
- **Omega-3 Fatty Acids & Biotin** – Help reduce scalp inflammation and strengthen hair.
- **Balanced Diet** – Include protein-rich foods, leafy greens, and anti-inflammatory nutrients.

4. **Scalp Care & Natural Remedies**

- **Essential Oils (Peppermint, Rosemary, Tea Tree)** – Improve circulation and reduce inflammation.
- **Aloe Vera & Neem Oil** – Help soothe an irritated scalp.
- **Scalp Massages** – Stimulate blood flow and promote healing.

5. **Professional Support**

- **Trichologists & Dermatologists** – Regular scalp assessments and biopsies can help determine the severity of CCCA and guide treatment.
- **Hair Restoration for Advanced Cases** – In severe scarring, hair transplants or scalp micropigmentation may be considered as potential solutions.

Final Thoughts

Central Centrifugal Cicatricial Alopecia (CCCA) is a progressive, scarring form of hair loss that disproportionately affects African American women. Since the damage can become permanent, early detection and proactive treatments are crucial. By modifying hair care practices, seeking medical treatments, and maintaining proper nutrition, individuals with CCCA can manage the condition effectively and preserve their hair health.

If you experience any early signs of CCCA, consult a dermatologist or trichologist for personalized advice and treatment options.

Traction Alopecia

Traction Alopecia (TA) is a preventable form of hair loss caused by continuous pulling or tension on the hair follicles. It most commonly affects the hairline, temples, and nape but can develop anywhere on the scalp subjected to excessive strain.

When detected early, hair regrowth is possible. However, if left untreated, repeated tension can lead to permanent follicular damage and scarring, making regrowth difficult or impossible.

Causes of Traction Alopecia

TA results from mechanical stress on the hair follicles due to various styling practices, accessories, and habitual pulling.

1. Tight Hairstyles & Protective Styles

While protective styles help maintain hair health, overly tight styles can cause long-term damage, including:

- Braids, cornrows, twists, and dreadlocks (especially when styled too tightly)
- High ponytails and buns that constantly pull on the scalp

- Weaves, sew-ins, and wigs secured with tight tracks or adhesives
- Micro-links and extensions that exert excessive strain on hair follicles

2. Hair Accessories & Styling Practices

- Tight elastic bands and hair ties that pull at the roots
- Frequent use of bobby pins and clips, especially when secured tightly
- Headbands or helmets that constantly rub against the scalp

3. Chemical & Heat Damage

- Chemical relaxers weaken the hair shaft, making it more prone to breakage under tension.
- Frequent heat styling (flat irons, curling wands) reduces hair elasticity, increasing the risk of tension-related damage.

4. Habitual Pulling & Manipulation

- Constantly twisting, tugging, or pulling hair (even unconsciously) stresses follicles over time.
- Trichotillomania, a psychological hair-pulling disorder, can exacerbate hair loss and increase the risk of permanent damage.

Symptoms of Traction Alopecia

Recognizing the early signs of TA is essential for preventing permanent damage.

Early Signs

- Hairline thinning, especially along the temples and edges
- Redness and scalp tenderness from constant pulling

- Small bumps (folliculitis) along the hairline, indicating irritated follicles
- Scalp soreness or itchiness, leading to discomfort when styling hair

Advanced Symptoms

- A receding hairline with noticeable thinning
- Bald patches from prolonged follicular stress
- A shiny or smooth scalp, indicating scarring that makes hair regrowth difficult

Solutions & Treatment for Traction Alopecia

1. Stop the Tension Immediately

- Loosen hairstyles to reduce scalp strain.
- Take breaks from continuous use of weaves, wigs, and braids.
- Use softer accessories like silk or satin scrunchies instead of tight elastics.

2. Encourage Hair Regrowth

- Scalp massages stimulate blood circulation and encourage follicle recovery.
- Essential oils (peppermint, rosemary, castor oil) promote hair regrowth.
- Topical Minoxidil (Rogaine 5%) can help if follicles are still viable.

3. Reduce Scalp Inflammation

- Aloe vera and neem oil soothe irritation and reduce inflammation.
- Corticosteroids, prescribed by a dermatologist, help control scalp inflammation and folliculitis.
- Antibiotics may be needed for infected follicles that develop pus-filled bumps.

4. Strengthen Hair & Prevent Further Damage

- Increase iron and vitamin D intake to support follicle health.
- Omega-3 fatty acids and biotin improve scalp health and help prevent breakage.
- Use gentle, sulfate-free hair products to maintain scalp moisture.

5. Protective Hairstyles Without Tension

- Loose twists, bantu knots, and braid-outs
- Low, loose ponytails instead of tight buns
- Clip-ins and glueless wigs instead of tight sewn-in weaves

6. Medical & Professional Interventions

- **Platelet-Rich Plasma (PRP) Therapy** – Injects growth factors into the scalp to stimulate hair regrowth.
- **Hair Transplant Surgery** – May be an option for severe scarring cases.

Preventing Traction Alopecia Long-Term

- Rotate hairstyles to avoid excessive tension on the same areas.
- Moisturize and condition hair regularly to prevent dryness and brittleness.
- Sleep on a silk or satin pillowcase or wear a satin scarf to reduce friction.
- Consult a trichologist or dermatologist at the first signs of hair loss.

Final Thoughts

Traction Alopecia is one of the most preventable types of hair loss. The key to stopping TA is early intervention, gentle styling, and healthy scalp care. By taking proactive steps—such as avoiding tight hairstyles, heat, and chemical damage—you can preserve your hairline and maintain healthy hair growth.

Seborrheic Dermatitis and Psoriasis

Seborrheic Dermatitis (SD) and Scalp Psoriasis are two common chronic scalp conditions that cause itching, flaking, and inflammation. While both can significantly affect scalp health and hair retention, they have distinct causes and treatments. Recognizing the differences is key to effective management and preventing hair loss.

Seborrheic Dermatitis (SD)

Seborrheic Dermatitis is a chronic inflammatory condition that affects the scalp, face, and other sebaceous (oil-producing) areas of the skin. It is often linked to an overgrowth of yeast (Malassezia), excessive sebum production, and an inflammatory response.

Causes of Seborrheic Dermatitis

- **Overproduction of Sebum** – Excess oil provides an ideal environment for Malassezia yeast to thrive.
- **Fungal Overgrowth (Malassezia)** – A naturally occurring yeast that can trigger inflammation in sensitive individuals.
- **Genetic Predisposition** – Family history plays a role in susceptibility to SD.
- **Environmental Factors** – Cold weather, humidity, and stress can worsen flare-ups.
- **Immune System Dysfunction** – More common in individuals with weakened immune systems.

Symptoms of Seborrheic Dermatitis

- Greasy, yellowish flakes or dandruff
- Itchy and inflamed scalp
- Red or irritated skin along the hairline, ears, and eyebrows
- Burning or stinging sensation
- Worsening with stress, seasonal changes, or poor scalp hygiene

Scalp Psoriasis

Scalp Psoriasis is an autoimmune condition that causes rapid skin cell turnover, leading to thick, scaly plaques. It can affect not only the scalp but also other areas of the body, such as the elbows, knees, and back.

Causes of Scalp Psoriasis

- **Genetics** – Psoriasis often runs in families.
- **Autoimmune Response** – The immune system mistakenly speeds up skin cell growth, forming thick scales.
- **Triggers** – Stress, infections, cold weather, and scalp injuries can cause flare-ups.

Symptoms of Scalp Psoriasis

- Thick, silvery-white scales or plaques
- Well-defined red patches covered with flaky skin
- Intense itching and burning
- Cracked or bleeding skin (in severe cases)
- May extend beyond the scalp to the neck and ears

Differences Between Seborrheic Dermatitis & Scalp Psoriasis

Feature	Seborrheic Dermatitis (SD)	Scalp Psoriasis
Flaking	Greasy, yellow flakes	Thick, silvery scales
Itching	Moderate to severe	Severe, may cause burning
Scalp Appearance	Red and inflamed	Well defined red patches
Cause	Malessezia yeast & oil production	Autoimmune response
Triggers	Stress, weather, oily scalp	Stress, infections, injury

Treatment & Management Strategies

For Seborrheic Dermatitis

1. **Anti-Dandruff & Antifungal Shampoos**

   - **Ketoconazole (Nizoral)** – Helps reduce Malassezia yeast.
   - **Selenium Sulfide (Selsun Blue)** – Controls flaking and inflammation.
   - **Zinc Pyrithione (Head & Shoulders Clinical)** – Fights fungal overgrowth.

2. **Scalp Cleansing & Hydration**

   - Wash hair **2-3 times per week** to minimize oil buildup.

- Use **sulfate-free shampoos** to prevent excessive dryness.
- **Diluted apple cider vinegar** rinses can help balance the scalp microbiome.

3. Soothing & Anti-Inflammatory Treatments

- **Aloe Vera, Tea Tree Oil, and Neem Oil** – Help reduce itching and inflammation.
- **Jojoba Oil** – Provides hydration without clogging pores.

4. Lifestyle Adjustments

- Manage stress levels to prevent flare-ups.
- Limit high-sugar and processed foods that contribute to inflammation.

For Scalp Psoriasis

1. Medical Shampoos & Topical Treatments

- **Coal Tar Shampoos** – Slow down excessive skin cell production.
- **Salicylic Acid Shampoos** – Help dissolve thick scales.
- **Steroid-Based Lotions (Prescribed)** – Reduce inflammation and scaling.

2. Scalp Moisturization

- Shea Butter, Aloe Vera, and Glycerin-based creams can soothe dryness.
- Avoid petroleum-based products, which may trap heat and worsen irritation.

3. Phototherapy & Prescription Medications

- **UVB Light Therapy** – Helps slow down excessive skin growth.

- **Biologic Injections or Oral Medications** – Used for severe cases.

4. **Avoid Triggers**

- Minimize alcohol consumption and processed foods.
- Keep the scalp moisturized to reduce flaking.
- Protect against harsh weather conditions with gentle head coverings.

Managing These Conditions in African American Hair Care

Gentle Hair Care Routine

- Avoid overwashing to maintain natural oils.

Protective Styling Without Tension

- Opt for loose braids, twists, or wigs that allow scalp airflow.

Oil-Based Scalp Treatments

- Use lightweight oils to prevent buildup and maintain hydration.

Regular Scalp Detox

- Herbal rinses, like rosemary or peppermint tea, can cleanse the scalp without harsh stripping.

When to See a Trichologist or Dermatologist

- If symptoms persist despite home treatments.
- If scalp sores, bleeding, or intense pain develop.
- If hair loss becomes noticeable or permanent patches appear.

Final Thoughts

Seborrheic Dermatitis and Scalp Psoriasis are chronic conditions that require consistent management to prevent discomfort and hair loss. While they share some similarities, understanding their differences allows for more targeted treatment.

If you're struggling with itching, flaking, or inflammation, making lifestyle changes, using medicated treatments, and adopting gentle hair care practices can help restore scalp health. For persistent or severe cases, consulting a dermatologist or trichologist is the best step toward long-term relief.

Fungal Infections (Tinea Capitis)

Tinea capitis, commonly known as scalp ringworm, is a contagious fungal infection that primarily affects children but can also occur in adults. It is caused by dermatophyte fungi such as *Trichophyton* and *Microsporum*, which thrive in warm, damp environments. The infection spreads through direct contact, contaminated objects, or infected animals, especially cats and dogs.

Causes & Risk Factors of Tinea Capitis

1. **Fungal Contamination**

   - Direct contact with an **infected person, pet, or contaminated surfaces**.
   - Sharing personal items like **combs, hats, pillows, and towels** increases the risk of infection.

2. **Warm, Humid Environments**

   - The fungus thrives in **sweaty scalps, damp conditions, and poor hygiene practices**.

3. **Weakened Immune System**

- Children, individuals with **compromised immunity**, and those with **nutritional deficiencies** are more susceptible.

4. Poor Scalp Hygiene & Occlusive Hairstyles

- Wearing **tight wigs, weaves, or braids** for extended periods can trap **moisture**, encouraging fungal overgrowth.

Symptoms of Tinea Capitis

Tinea capitis presents in **different stages**, from **mild scaling** to **severe inflammation and hair loss**.

Early Symptoms

- Round, **scaly patches** on the scalp.
- Itching and mild **redness**.
- **Dry, brittle hair** that breaks easily.
- **Flaking** that resembles dandruff.

Progressive Symptoms

- Patchy **hair loss** with **black dots** where hair shafts break at the scalp.
- **Painful, inflamed lesions (kerions)**—severe infections may cause swollen, pus-filled bumps.
- **Tender, swollen lymph nodes** near the ears and neck.
- **Crusting and oozing lesions**—if untreated, secondary **bacterial infections** may develop.

Treatment for Tinea Capitis

Tinea capitis requires medical treatment, as over-the-counter solutions alone are not effective.

1. Prescription Oral Antifungal Medications

- **Griseofulvin** – The most commonly prescribed antifungal (typically for 6–8 weeks).
- **Terbinafine (Lamisil)** – Another effective oral antifungal.
- **Itraconazole or Fluconazole** – May be used in resistant cases.

2. **Antifungal Shampoos (Adjunct Treatment)**

   - **Ketoconazole (Nizoral)** – Helps reduce fungal spores and prevent spread.
   - **Selenium Sulfide (Selsun Blue Medicated)** – Reduces fungal load and inflammation.
   - **Zinc Pyrithione (Head & Shoulders Clinical)** – Helps relieve scaling and flaking.

How to Use:

- Medicated shampoos should be used 2–3 times per week alongside oral antifungal medication for best results.

3. **Home Remedies (Supportive Care, Not a Cure)**

   - **Apple Cider Vinegar Rinse** – Contains natural antifungal properties to soothe the scalp.
   - **Tea Tree Oil (Diluted)** – Helps reduce itching and fungal overgrowth.
   - **Aloe Vera & Coconut Oil** – May aid scalp healing after treatment.

4. **Hygiene & Prevention**

   - Avoid sharing personal items such as combs, hats, and pillowcases.
   - Wash bedding, hats, and hair tools in hot water to eliminate fungal spores.
   - Check pets for signs of ringworm (patchy fur loss, scaly skin).

- Screen family members if they have been in close contact with an infected individual.

Preventing Recurrence

- Keep the scalp **clean and dry**—wash hair regularly to prevent fungal buildup.
- Avoid **tight hairstyles, occlusive wigs, or prolonged moisture buildup** that encourage fungal growth.
- Strengthen immunity with a **balanced diet rich in zinc, vitamin D, and antioxidants**.
- Monitor scalp health and seek early treatment to prevent severe hair loss.

When to See a Doctor

- If patchy hair loss or scalp swelling occurs.
- If kerions (painful, pus-filled sores) develop.
- If symptoms persist despite using antifungal shampoo.
- If a child in close contact with an infected individual develops similar symptoms

Contact Dermatitis

Contact dermatitis is an inflammatory skin reaction triggered by exposure to irritants or allergens. On the scalp, it is often caused by harsh chemicals in hair dyes, shampoos, relaxers, and styling products.

Types of Contact Dermatitis

1. Irritant Contact Dermatitis (ICD)

- Caused by **direct irritation** from substances like harsh shampoos and relaxers.

- Symptoms appear **immediately or within hours** of exposure.

2. Allergic Contact Dermatitis (ACD)

- Caused by an **immune system reaction** to allergens such as hair dye or preservatives.
- Symptoms may take **24–48 hours** to appear after exposure.

Common Causes & Triggers

- **Hair Dyes** (*p-Phenylenediamine (PPD), Ammonia, Resorcinol*).
- **Relaxers & Perms** (*Lye, Sodium Hydroxide, Thioglycolates*).
- **Shampoos & Conditioners** (*Sulfates, Parabens, Artificial Fragrances, Formaldehyde*).
- **Styling Products** (*Alcohol, Synthetic Fragrances, Preservatives*).
- **Essential Oils** (*Tea Tree, Peppermint—potential triggers for sensitive individuals*).

Symptoms of Contact Dermatitis on the Scalp

- **Redness & Inflammation** – The scalp appears swollen, red, and irritated.
- **Itching & Burning** – Often intense, leading to scratching and potential infections.
- **Dry, Flaky Patches** – May resemble dandruff or psoriasis-like scaling.
- **Blisters or Oozing Lesions** – Occur in severe allergic reactions.
- **Swelling Around the Scalp, Face, or Eyes** – Common in PPD allergies.

- **Hair Shedding or Breakage** – Due to scalp inflammation and follicle stress.

Treatment & Management

1. Remove the Irritant or Allergen

- Discontinue the offending product immediately.
- Wash the scalp with a gentle, sulfate-free shampoo.
- Avoid harsh styling products until the scalp fully heals.

2. Soothe the Scalp

- Apply a cold compress or aloe vera gel to reduce itching and inflammation.
- Use rosemary oil, neem oil, or chamomile extract for their natural anti-inflammatory effects.
- Consider topical hydrocortisone or antihistamines for severe itching.

3. Medications (For Severe Cases)

- **Oral Antihistamines** (*Benadryl, Zyrtec*) to calm allergic reactions.
- **Topical Steroids** (prescribed by a doctor) to reduce severe inflammation.
- **Antibiotics** may be necessary if a secondary bacterial infection develops.

4. Scalp Recovery & Strengthening

- Use a sulfate-free, fragrance-free shampoo (*e.g., Vanicream, Free & Clear*).
- Apply a gentle scalp serum with ceramides or hyaluronic acid for hydration.
- Massage the scalp lightly to promote circulation without aggravating irritation.

Preventing Future Reactions

- **Patch Test New Products** – Apply a small amount behind the ear and wait **48 hours** before full use.
- **Choose Hypoallergenic Hair Care** – Look for **PPD-free, ammonia-free, and sulfate-free** formulations.
- **Limit Chemical Treatments** – Opt for gentler, plant-based hair dyes or natural styling alternatives.
- **Avoid Excessive Heat & Styling** – Irritated skin is more prone to damage.
- **Keep the Scalp Moisturized** – Dry, compromised skin is more reactive to allergens.

When to See a Doctor

- If the reaction does not improve within a few days.
- If there is severe swelling, pain, or oozing blisters.
- If hair loss becomes noticeable or permanent.

Final Thoughts

Contact dermatitis of the scalp can be both painful and frustrating, but early identification and avoiding triggers are key to preventing recurrence. Using gentle, hypoallergenic hair care products and maintaining good scalp hygiene can help keep the scalp healthy and reduce flare-ups. If symptoms persist or worsen, seeking medical advice is essential for effective treatment and long-term scalp health.

Underlying Causes and Risk Factors

Hair loss and scalp conditions do not stem from a single cause but rather result from a combination of genetic, structural, cultural, and nutritional factors. Understanding these underlying causes is essential for effectively preventing and managing hair and scalp issues.

1. Genetic Factors and Hair Loss

Genetics play a significant role in hair density, growth cycles, and susceptibility to scalp conditions. Certain forms of hair loss, such as alopecia areata (AA), central centrifugal cicatricial alopecia (CCCA), and androgenetic alopecia (AGA), are strongly linked to genetic predisposition.

Alopecia Areata (AA) & Genetics

- An autoimmune-related condition where the immune system attacks hair follicles.
- More common in individuals with a family history of autoimmune diseases (e.g., lupus, rheumatoid arthritis).
- Linked to specific HLA gene variations, which increase susceptibility.

Central Centrifugal Cicatricial Alopecia (CCCA) & Genetics

- More prevalent among African American women.
- Studies suggest inherited inflammatory responses contribute to follicular scarring and destruction.
- Associated with mutations in the *PADI3* gene, which affects hair shaft integrity.

Androgenetic Alopecia (AGA) & Genetics

- The **most common** cause of hair loss in both **men and women**.
- Sensitivity to dihydrotestosterone (DHT) leads to follicular miniaturization and progressive hair thinning.
- A family history of male or female pattern baldness increases the risk.

2. Hair Structure & Its Impact on Fragility

Hair texture and structure influence its susceptibility to damage, particularly in individuals with Afro-textured hair.

Unique Characteristics of African American Hair

- **Thinner Cuticle Layer**

    - The outer protective layer is naturally thinner, making it more vulnerable to friction, styling damage, and chemicals.

- **Asymmetric Follicle Growth**

    - Curly hair grows from oval or asymmetrical follicles, resulting in a twisting pattern that makes strands weaker and more prone to breakage.

- **Higher Prone to Mechanical Damage**

    - The tight curl pattern leads to tangling and knotting, increasing shedding and breakage during detangling.

Implications of Hair Structure on Scalp Health

- Sebum (natural scalp oil) has difficulty traveling down the hair shaft, leading to dryness, brittleness, and breakage.

- Moisture retention challenges require hydration-focused hair care routines to maintain hair strength and flexibility.

3. Cultural Hair Care Practices & Their Effects

Both traditional and modern hair care practices play a crucial role in maintaining hair health. However, certain habits can contribute to hair loss and scalp conditions if not managed properly.

Chemical Relaxers & Hair Straightening Treatments

Chemical Relaxers (Lye & No-Lye Formulas)

- Contain sodium hydroxide (lye) or calcium hydroxide (no-lye), which break down hair proteins to straighten curls.
- Overuse can lead to thinning, breakage, scalp burns, and follicular damage.
- Linked to scarring alopecia (CCCA) and chronic scalp inflammation.

Brazilian Keratin Treatments (Formaldehyde-based Treatments)

- Contain formaldehyde, a toxic chemical known to cause scalp irritation, hair thinning, and breakage.
- Prolonged use weakens follicles, contributing to increased shedding.

Heat Styling (Flat Irons, Curling Wands, Blow Drying)

- Excessive heat exposure causes moisture loss, protein breakdown, and heat damage.
- Repeated use weakens hair shafts, leading to split ends and brittleness.

Protective Styles: Pros & Cons

Protective styles such as braids, weaves, wigs, and locs help reduce daily manipulation but can also cause scalp stress if not maintained properly.

Benefits of Protective Styles

- Low manipulation reduces breakage.
- Helps retain length by minimizing friction.
- Shields hair from environmental damage.

Potential Risks of Protective Styles

- Tight braids & ponytails → Can cause traction alopecia.
- Weaves & wigs → May lead to scalp buildup and fungal growth if not properly maintained.
- Glue-based applications → Can cause hairline damage and follicular stress.

Solution

- Rotate styles and avoid excessive tension.
- Prioritize scalp hydration and cleansing.

4. Nutritional Deficiencies & Their Impact on Hair Health

Nutrients play a critical role in hair growth and follicular health. Deficiencies in key vitamins and minerals can contribute to increased hair loss and scalp conditions.

Key Nutrients for Hair Health

Vitamin D

- Essential for follicle cycling and immune regulation.
- Deficiency is linked to hair thinning and alopecia areata.
- **Sources:** Sun exposure, fatty fish, fortified dairy, mushrooms.

Iron (Ferritin Levels)

- Low iron levels can cause Telogen Effluvium (excessive shedding).
- Essential for red blood cell oxygenation, which nourishes the scalp.
- **Sources:** Red meat, spinach, lentils, fortified cereals.

Zinc

- Regulates sebum production and supports immune function.
- Deficiency can lead to brittle hair, increased shedding, and slower growth.
- **Sources:** Nuts, seeds, seafood, eggs, whole grains.

Omega-3 Fatty Acids

- Helps maintain scalp hydration and reduces inflammation.
- Essential for preventing dryness, dandruff, and scalp conditions like psoriasis.
- **Sources:** Salmon, flaxseeds, walnuts, chia seeds.

Biotin (Vitamin B7) & Other B-Complex Vitamins

- Supports keratin production and strengthens hair strands.
- Deficiency can cause hair thinning, brittleness, and slow regrowth.
- **Sources:** Eggs, nuts, whole grains, bananas.

Addressing These Risk Factors for Healthier Hair

1. Genetic Awareness

- If you have a family history of hair loss, start scalp care early.

- Consider **DHT blockers** for androgenetic alopecia (AGA) or **anti-inflammatory treatments** for central centrifugal cicatricial alopecia (CCCA).

2. Adjust Hair Care Practices

- Use **gentle, sulfate-free shampoos** to cleanse the scalp without stripping moisture.
- Opt for **low-heat styling** methods to minimize hair damage.
- Avoid **tight hairstyles** and excessive scalp tension.

3. Balanced Nutrition

- Increase intake of **iron, vitamin D, and omega-3s** to support hair health.
- Stay hydrated for optimal scalp function.

4. Scalp & Hair Strengthening Regimen

- Regular scalp massages with essential oils (rosemary, peppermint, castor oil) improve circulation.
- Deep condition weekly to combat dryness and strengthen strands.
- Limit chemical treatments and allow the scalp time to recover.

Final Thoughts

Hair loss and scalp issues arise from multiple factors, including genetics, hair structure, cultural hair care practices, and nutrition. A **holistic approach**—incorporating gentle hair care, balanced nutrition, and early intervention—can help preserve hair health and prevent unnecessary hair loss.

By understanding these risk factors, individuals can make **informed decisions** about their hair care routines, styling choices, and dietary habits to maintain healthy, resilient hair. If hair loss becomes persistent, consulting a

dermatologist or trichologist is recommended for personalized treatment and care.

Diagnostic Approaches

Accurate diagnosis is crucial for identifying the underlying causes of hair loss, inflammation, and scalp disorders. Trichologists and dermatologists use a combination of visual assessments, trichoscopic imaging, microscopic analysis, and laboratory tests to pinpoint specific conditions and recommend targeted treatments.

1. Visual and Physical Examination

A thorough scalp examination is the first step in diagnosing hair and scalp conditions. This process helps identify visible patterns of hair loss, inflammation, and follicular health issues.

Key Assessments During Physical Examination:

Assessing Hair Loss Patterns

- **Diffuse thinning** – Suggests telogen effluvium or androgenetic alopecia (AGA).
- **Patchy bald spots** – Indicates alopecia areata, traction alopecia, or scarring conditions.
- **Crown-centered thinning** – Common in **central centrifugal cicatricial alopecia (CCCA)** or female-pattern hair loss.

Examining Scalp Health

- **Redness and inflammation** – Seen in seborrheic dermatitis, psoriasis, or allergic reactions.
- **Scaling or flaking** – Suggests dandruff, fungal infections (tinea capitis), or psoriasis.
- **Pain, tenderness, or burning** – May indicate inflammatory conditions like CCCA or lichen planopilaris.

- **Oozing, crusting, or pustules** – Can signal bacterial or fungal infections.

Hair Shaft and Follicle Condition

- **Broken hair shafts** – Common in traction alopecia, chemical damage, or trichotillomania.
- **Short, stubby hairs (exclamation mark hairs)** – Indicative of alopecia areata.
- **Perifollicular scaling and follicular plugging** – Common in scarring alopecias.

A physical exam helps narrow down possible conditions before proceeding to advanced diagnostic tools.

2. Trichoscopic Evaluation (Trichoscopy)

Trichoscopy is a non-invasive imaging technique that magnifies the hair and scalp up to 100–200 times, providing detailed visualization of follicular and scalp structures.

Advantages of Trichoscopy

- Differentiates between scarring and non-scarring hair loss.
- Detects early-stage hair disorders before significant shedding occurs.
- Helps monitor treatment progress over time.

3. Microscopic Analysis

Microscopic examination of hair and scalp samples allows for the assessment of hair bulb and shaft abnormalities, as well as fungal infections, at a cellular level.

Types of Microscopic Tests

Bright-Field Microscopy

- Identifies hair shaft abnormalities such as trichorrhexis nodosa, monilethrix, and pili torti.

- Detects hair breakage patterns caused by mechanical damage or chemical overuse.

Polarized Light Dermoscopy

- Detects structural abnormalities in the hair shaft.
- Identifies excess keratin buildup, cuticle damage, or pigment defects.

Fungal Culture & Direct Microscopic Examination (KOH Test)

- Potassium hydroxide (KOH) preparation detects fungal spores in tinea capitis.
- Fungal cultures confirm the exact fungal strain for targeted antifungal treatment.

4. Additional Diagnostic Tests

Hair Pull Test (For Active Shedding Conditions)

- A gentle tug of 60 hairs from different scalp areas is performed.
- If more than 10% of hairs are shed, it suggests an active hair shedding disorder such as telogen effluvium or alopecia areata.

Hair Pluck Test (For Root Analysis)

- Hairs are plucked from different areas and examined under a microscope.
- Helps determine whether the hair is in the anagen (growth), catagen (transition), or telogen (shedding) phase.

Scalp Biopsy (For Severe or Scarring Cases)

- A small scalp tissue sample is taken for histological examination.
- Helps diagnose scarring alopecias like CCCA, lichen planopilaris (LPP), and frontal fibrosing alopecia.

- Can confirm autoimmune or inflammatory scalp conditions.

Blood Tests (For Nutritional & Hormonal Imbalances)

Test	Purpose
Ferritin (Iron Levels)	Low levels linked to diffuse hair thinning.
Vitamin D & Zinc Levels	Essential for healthy follicular function
Thyroid Panel (TSH, T3, T4)	Hypothyroidism can cause excessive shedding
Hormone Tests (DHEA, Androgens, Estrogen, Testosterone)	Helps identify hormonal-related hair loss (PCOS, AGA)

5. Choosing the Right Diagnostic Approach

Condition	Recommended Tests
Androgenetic Alopecia (AGA)	Trichoscopy, Hair Pull Test, Hormonal Blood Tests
Alopecia Areata (AA)	Trichoscopy, Hair Pluck Test, Scalp Biopsy
CCCA	Trichoscopy, Scalp Biopsy
Seborrheic Dermatitis	Visual Exam, Trichoscopy
Psoriasis	Trichoscopy, Visual Exam
Tinea Capitis (Fungal Infection)	KOH Test, Fungal Culture, Microscopy
Telogen Effluvium (TE)	Hair Pull Test, Blood Tests (Iron, Thyroid

Conclusion

An accurate diagnosis is crucial for effectively treating hair loss and scalp conditions. By combining visual examination, trichoscopy, microscopic analysis, and laboratory tests, specialists can gain a comprehensive understanding of scalp health and determine the most appropriate treatment options.

If hair loss or scalp symptoms persist, consulting a trichologist or dermatologist ensures a precise diagnosis and proper management of the condition.

Treatment and Management Strategies

Managing hair and scalp conditions requires a comprehensive approach that includes preventive measures, medical interventions, and holistic strategies. A personalized plan can help prevent further damage, promote hair regrowth, and maintain overall scalp health.

1. Preventive Measures

Education and proactive care are essential for preventing scalp issues and maintaining healthy hair growth.

Safe Styling Practices

- Avoid tight hairstyles (e.g., braids, ponytails, weaves) that cause traction alopecia and scalp tension. Opt for looser, low-manipulation styles.
- Minimize heat exposure from flat irons, curling wands, and blow dryers, as excessive heat weakens hair strands, leading to breakage and thinning. Always use a heat protectant.
- Use protective styles with caution to ensure they do not pull on the scalp or hinder proper hygiene.

Choosing the Right Hair Care Products

- Use sulfate-free, gentle shampoos to prevent dryness and irritation.
- Avoid harsh chemicals found in relaxers, ammonia-based dyes, and formaldehyde-containing treatments, which can cause scalp inflammation and breakage.
- Maintain hydration and scalp health by deep conditioning weekly with ingredients like aloe vera, shea butter, and hyaluronic acid.

Scalp Cleansing & Hygiene

- Wash hair 1–2 times per week to prevent buildup while retaining moisture.
- Use scalp exfoliants like salicylic acid or apple cider vinegar to remove dead skin and reduce dandruff.
- Apply essential oils (tea tree, rosemary, peppermint) to reduce inflammation and promote circulation.

2. Medical Interventions

For moderate to severe hair and scalp conditions, topical, injectable, and systemic treatments may be necessary.

Corticosteroids for Inflammatory Conditions

- Intralesional corticosteroid injections treat CCCA, alopecia areata, and lichen planopilaris, reducing inflammation and slowing hair loss.
- Topical corticosteroids (e.g., Clobetasol, Betamethasone) help manage scalp psoriasis, seborrheic dermatitis, and inflammatory scalp disorders.

Hair Growth Stimulants & Scalp Treatments

- **Minoxidil (Rogaine 5%)** is FDA-approved for **androgenetic alopecia**, stimulating follicular regrowth.
- **Oral Finasteride & Dutasteride** (for AGA in men) block **DHT**, slowing genetic hair loss progression.
- **Calcineurin inhibitors** (Tacrolimus, Pimecrolimus) serve as steroid alternatives for scalp inflammation and autoimmune conditions.

Antifungal & Antibacterial Treatments

- **Ketoconazole shampoo (Nizoral)** treats seborrheic dermatitis and fungal infections (e.g., tinea capitis).
- **Oral antibiotics** (e.g., Clindamycin, Doxycycline) treat folliculitis, scalp infections, or inflamed scarring alopecias.
- **Oral antifungals** (e.g., Griseofulvin, Terbinafine) are used for resistant fungal infections.

Scalp Procedures & Advanced Therapies

- **Platelet-Rich Plasma (PRP) Therapy** stimulates dormant follicles using growth factors from the patient's blood.
- **Hair transplants** are an option for severe androgenetic alopecia or scarring alopecia.
- **Low-Level Laser Therapy (LLLT)** enhances cellular energy production in follicles, improving hair density over time.

Referral to a dermatologist or trichologist is recommended for severe or unresponsive cases.

3. Holistic Approaches

A natural, lifestyle-based approach supports scalp health and hair regrowth.

Scalp & Hair Strengthening with Natural Oils

- **Jojoba oil** mimics natural scalp sebum, preventing dryness.
- **Castor oil** contains **ricinoleic acid**, which improves blood circulation and promotes growth.
- **Rosemary & peppermint oils** have been shown to stimulate hair growth and improve scalp circulation.

Nutrition & Diet for Hair Growth

A nutrient-dense diet supports healthy hair follicles and reduces hair loss risk.

- **Protein (Keratin Production)** – Eggs, fish, chicken, lentils, nuts.
- **Iron (Prevents Shedding)** – Spinach, red meat, and beans.
- **Omega-3 Fatty Acids (Scalp Hydration & Anti-Inflammatory Benefits)** –Salmon, flaxseeds, walnuts.
- **Vitamin C (Collagen Production & Iron Absorption)** – Citrus fruits, bell peppers.
- **Biotin & B-Complex Vitamins (Hair Strengthening)** – Avocados, whole grains, eggs.
- **Vitamin D (Follicular Growth)** – Sun exposure, fortified dairy, and mushrooms.

Diet Tips:

- Stay hydrated to keep the scalp moisturized.

- Reduce processed foods and sugar, which contribute to inflammation and hair thinning.

4. Stress Management & Scalp Stimulation

Chronic stress contributes to **telogen effluvium** (excessive shedding) and autoimmune hair loss conditions.

- **Meditation & deep breathing** lower cortisol levels, reducing stress-induced hair loss.
- **Scalp massages** using fingertips or a scalp massager improve circulation and follicle health.
- **Regular exercise** boosts oxygen supply to the scalp, promoting healthy hair growth cycles.

Final Thoughts: A Personalized Approach

- Prevent damage with gentle styling, moisture retention, and sulfate-free products.
- Use medical treatments like corticosteroids, Minoxidil, or antifungals when necessary.
- Support regrowth naturally with oils, scalp massages, and a nutrient-rich diet.
- Manage stress to prevent excessive shedding and inflammation.

By combining preventive care, medical intervention, and holistic strategies, individuals can effectively manage hair and scalp conditions while promoting long-term scalp health and hair growth. If hair loss or scalp irritation persists, consulting a dermatologist or trichologist is recommended for a comprehensive evaluation and personalized treatment plan.

Conclusion

Maintaining healthy hair and scalp requires a comprehensive approach that considers the unique structural, cultural, and environmental factors affecting African American individuals. Understanding genetic predispositions, hair structure, styling practices, and common scalp conditions allows individuals to take proactive steps toward prevention, treatment, and long-term hair care solutions.

By combining scientific research with culturally informed practices, trichologists and hair care professionals can develop personalized strategies that promote scalp health and hair growth while empowering individuals to embrace their natural hair and effectively address concerns that may arise.

Key Takeaways

1. Preventive Care is Essential

- Educating individuals on gentle styling, proper hydration, and avoiding harsh treatments is key to preventing hair loss and scalp disorders.

2. Medical Interventions & Holistic Approaches Work Together

- Combining topical treatments, medical solutions, and natural scalp care yields optimal results for various hair and scalp conditions.

3. Nutritional Health & Stress Management Play a Role

- A well-balanced diet rich in essential vitamins and minerals, along with effective stress management, supports stronger, healthier hair and reduces shedding.

4. Trichoscopic & Microscopic Diagnostics Provide Early Detection

- Advanced scalp imaging, trichoscopy, and lab tests help identify hair loss conditions before irreversible damage occurs, allowing for timely intervention.

5. Empowerment Through Education & Advocacy

- Promoting ongoing research, awareness, and culturally sensitive hair care education fosters long-term improvements in hair health and maintenance.

This guide serves as a foundational resource for African American hair and scalp health, integrating scientific research, practical experience, and holistic solutions to support sustainable, effective treatment plans. With the right knowledge and care, individuals can achieve healthy, thriving hair while preserving the integrity of their natural texture.

QUIZ
UNDERSTANDING AND ADDRESSING AFRICAN AMERICAN HAIR AND SCALP HEALTH

1. Question

What is the primary symptom that distinguishes Central Centrifugal Cicatricial Alopecia (CCCA) from other types of hair loss?

a) Hair loss starting from the hairline.

b) Red patches on the scalp.

c) Hair loss beginning at the crown and progressing outward.

d) Greasy yellow flakes throughout the scalp.

Answer: c) Hair loss beginning at the crown and progressing outward.

2. Question

Which of the following is a key cause of traction alopecia?

a) Nutritional deficiency.

b) Excessive sun exposure.

c) Chronic tight hairstyles and mechanical stress.

d) Fungal infections.

Answer: c) Chronic tight hairstyles and mechanical stress.

3. Question

Which ingredient in chemical hair dyes is a common allergen and cause of contact dermatitis?

a) Zinc Pyrithione

b) Ketoconazole

c) p-Phenylenediamine (PPD)

d) Salicylic Acid

Answer: c) p-Phenylenediamine (PPD)

4. Question

Which of the following nutrients plays a key role in preventing scalp inflammation and promoting hydration?

a) Vitamin C

b) Zinc

c) Omega-3 fatty acids

d) Calcium

Answer: c) Omega-3 fatty acids

5. Question

Which tool is most commonly used to non-invasively examine scalp and follicle structure in detail?

a) Hair pull test

b) Trichoscopy

c) Bright-field microscopy

d) Hair pluck test

Answer: b) Trichoscopy

6. Question

Which scalp condition is associated with thick, silvery plaques and may extend beyond the scalp?

a) Seborrheic Dermatitis

b) Tinea Capitis

c) Scalp Psoriasis

d) Contact Dermatitis

Answer: c) Scalp Psoriasis

7. Question

What is the most effective first-line treatment for tinea capitis?

a) Topical tea tree oil

b) Coal tar shampoo

c) Oral antifungal medication

d) Hydrocortisone cream

Answer: c) Oral antifungal medication

8. Question

Which of the following structural features contributes to increased fragility in African American hair?

a) Round follicles and thick cuticle.

b) Symmetrical follicle growth.

c) Thinner cuticle layer and asymmetrical follicle shape.

d) Excessive sebum production.

Answer: c) Thinner cuticle layer and asymmetrical follicle shape.

9. Question

Which of the following is an appropriate holistic practice to support scalp circulation and follicle health?

a) Dry brushing the scalp.

b) Daily tight buns.

c) Scalp massages with essential oils.

d) Using alcohol-based astringents.

Answer: c) Scalp massages with essential oils.

10. Question

Which diagnostic test would most likely confirm a fungal scalp infection such as tinea capitis?

a) Ferritin blood test

b) KOH test and fungal culture

c) Scalp biopsy

d) Hormone panel

Answer: b) KOH test and fungal culture

CLOSING NOTE

Healing your scalp is an act of love.

It's permission to rest, restore, and reconnect with the parts of yourself that have been overlooked. You deserve relief—and you deserve regrowth.

www.ingramcontent.com/pod-product-compliance
Lightning Source LLC
Chambersburg PA
CBHW052143270326
41930CB00012B/2995